Table of Contents

Alzheimer's disease is a brain disorder that slowly destroys memory and thinking skills and, eventually, and the ability to carry out the simplest tasks. In most people with the disease — those with the late-onset type symptoms first appear in their mid-60s. Early-onset Alzheimer's occurs between a person's 30s and mid-60s and is very rare. Alzheimer's disease is the most common cause of dementia among older adults.

Understanding types of dementia

Share this infographic and help spread the word about understanding different types of dementia.

The disease is named after Dr. Alois Alzheimer. In 1906, Dr. Alzheimer noticed changes in the brain tissue of a woman who had died of an unusual mental illness. Her symptoms included memory loss, language problems, and unpredictable behavior. After she died, he examined her brain and found many abnormal clumps (now called amyloid plaques) and tangled bundles of fibers (now called neurofibrillary, or tau, tangles).

These plaques and tangles in the brain are still considered some of the main features of Alzheimer's disease. Another feature is the loss of connections between nerve cells (neurons) in the brain. Neurons transmit messages between different parts of the brain, and from the brain to muscles and organs in the body. Many other complex brain changes are thought to play a role in Alzheimer's, too.

This damage initially takes place in parts of the brain involved in memory, including the entorhinal cortex and hippocampus. It later affects areas in the cerebral cortex, such as those responsible for language, reasoning, and social behavior. Eventually, many other areas of the brain are damaged.

BREAKFAST

1. Best Chocolate Chip Cookies

Prep Time: 10 Minutes

Cook Time: 11 Minutes

Servings: 12

Ingredients

- 2 cups all-purpose flour 240 grams
- 1.5 ounces instant maple and brown sugar oatmeal 43 grams (1 package)
- 1 teaspoon baking soda 6 grams
- ½ teaspoon kosher salt
- ½ teaspoon cornstarch
- ½ cup unsalted butter 113 grams, room temperature (1 stick)
- 1½ cups brown sugar 320 grams
- ¼ cup granulated sugar 50 grams
- 2 large eggs 100 grams, room temperature
- 1 teaspoon pure vanilla extract 4 grams
- 2 tablespoons half-and-half 28 grams
- 1 cup semisweet chocolate chips 170 grams

Instructions

1. Preheat oven 375°F. Line a baking sheet with parchment paper. Set aside.

2. In a small bowl, mix the flour, oatmeal, baking soda, salt, and cornstarch. Set aside

3. 2 cups all-purpose flour, 1.5 ounces instant maple and brown sugar oatmeal, 1 teaspoon baking soda, ½ teaspoon kosher salt, ½ teaspoon cornstarch

4. Flour in a clear glass bowl

5. Place the butter, brown sugar, and sugar in a large bowl. Using a hand mixer, cream them together. Add the eggs, vanilla, and half-and-half. Whisk well to combine

6. ½ cup unsalted butter,1½ cups brown sugar,¼ cup granulated sugar,2 large eggs,1 teaspoon pure vanilla extract,2 tablespoons half-and-half

7. Dough in a mixing bowl

8. Add the flour mix to the wet mix and beat on medium speed for 10 seconds

9. Making the best chocolate chip cookies

10. Fold the chocolate chips into the cookie dough

11. 1 cup semisweet chocolate chips

12. bowl of raw cookie dough

13. Form 1-inch balls using a cookie portion scoop or a spoon

14. Place the cookies onto the prepared baking sheet. Using a spatula, lightly press the top of the cookie dough to flatten.

15. Uncooked Cooke dough on a baking sheet

16. Bake for 11 minutes. Serve warm with milk and enjoy!

Prep Time: 15 Minutes

Cook Time: 10 Minutes

Servings: 10

Ingredients

- 1 tablespoon olive oil
- 1/2 pound cooked chicken shredded (I used cooked Rotisserie chicken)
- 1 ounce Taco Seasoning click for homemade recipe!
- 1/2 cup onion diced
- 1 can diced tomato 14.5 ounce, fully drained
- 1 can Chopped Green Chiles 4.5 ounce, fully drained
- 10 Stand and Stuff Taco Shells I used Old El Paso
- 8 ounces Refried Beans 1/2 can
- 2 cups Mexican Blend Cheese shredded
- Toppings such as Old El Paso sliced Jalapenos, sour cream, salsa, chopped cilantro, shredded lettuce, or any of your favorite taco toppings!

Instructions

1. Preheat oven to 400F. Spray a 9×13 baking dish with nonstick spray.
2. Heat olive oil over medium heat in a medium skillet.
3. Add onion to skillet and cook for 2-3 minutes, or until the onion is translucent and fragrant.
4. Stir in the chicken, taco seasoning, tomatoes (FULLY DRAINED), and green chiles (FULLY DRAINED) see

     note. Stir to combine fully. Reduce to simmer and allow to cook for 5-8 minutes.

5. Place the taco shells in the baking dish, standing up. I was able to fit 10 taco shells in the dish by adding 2 on each side.
6. Bake the taco shells for 5 minutes by themselves to allow them to crisp up. Remove from the oven.
7. Spoon 1 tablespoon of beans into the bottom of each taco shell. Top with the chicken mixture, almost to the top of each shell.
8. Sprinkle each shell generously with shredded cheese, the more the better!
9. Bake for 7-10 minutes or until cheese is fully melted and the edges of the shells are browned.
10. Remove from the oven and top with your favorite items such as jalapenos, sour cream, cilantro, and salsa.
11. Enjoy!

Prep Time: 15 Minutes

Cook Time: 15 Minutes

Servings: 24

Ingredients

- 1 cup unsalted butter 226 grams, room temperature (2 sticks)
- 1 cup dark brown sugar 213 grams
- ½ cup granulated sugar 100 grams
- 2 large eggs 100 grams, room temperature
- 2 teaspoons pure vanilla extract 8 grams
- 1¼ cups Bob's Red Mill Unbleached White All-Purpose Flour 204 grams
- ½ teaspoon Bob's Red Mill Baking Soda 3 grams
- 1 teaspoon kosher salt 3 grams
- 3 cups Bob's Red Mill Old Fashioned Rolled Oats 300 grams
- 2 cups semisweet chocolate chips 340 grams

Instructions

1. Preheat oven to 325°F. Line a baking sheet with parchment paper and set aside.
2. Using an electric hand mixer, beat the butter, brown sugar, and sugar together until light and fluffy, about 3 minutes. Scrape down the sides as needed.
3. 1 cup unsalted butter, 1 cup dark brown sugar, ½ cup granulated sugar
4. how to make oatmeal chocolate chip cookies

5. Add in the eggs and mix until combined. Add in the vanilla and mix again. Set aside.
6. 2 large eggs, 2 teaspoons pure vanilla extract
7. In a medium bowl, whisk the flour, baking soda, and salt together.
8. 1¼ cups Bob's Red Mill Unbleached White All-Purpose Flour, ½ teaspoon Bob's Red Mill Baking Soda,1 teaspoon kosher salt
9. how to make oatmeal chocolate chip cookies
10. Add the dry ingredients to the wet ingredients and mix until just combined.
11. how to make oatmeal chocolate chip cookies
12. Fold in the oats and chocolate chips.
13. 3 cups Bob's Red Mill Old Fashioned Rolled Oats, 2 cups semisweet chocolate chips
14. how to make oatmeal chocolate chip cookies
15. Using a large cookie scoop (about ¼ cup), scoop the dough onto the prepared sheet pan, leaving 2 inches between the cookies.
16. how to make oatmeal chocolate chip cookies
17. Bake for 14-18 minutes until the edges of the cookies are golden and the centers are set. Let cool on the sheet pan for 3 minutes. Transfer to a wire rack to cool.

Prep Time: 5 Minutes

Cook Time: 15 Minutes

Servings: 8

Ingredients

- 12 ounces evaporated milk (1 can)
- 1 tablespoon cornstarch
- 3/4 lb white American cheese buy it sliced at the deli counter at your grocery store. Then chop into small squares, finely chopped
- 4 ounces mozzarella cheese shredded
- 2 tablespoons canned jalapenos chopped, or chopped green chiles
- 1 teaspoon chili powder you could also use cumin if you prefer that taste
- 1/2 teaspoon ground nutmeg optional. Some readers haven't liked this spice although some did,
- 1 teaspoon red pepper flakes
- 1/4 teaspoon salt
- 1/4 teaspoon black pepper
- chopped cilantro tomatoes, and jalapenos for garnish

Instructions

1. Heat evaporated milk over medium/high heat in a small saucepan. Stir in the cornstarch and whisk to combine.

2. Once simmering (bring to JUST before boil…when it starts bubbling up the sides its ready), reduce heat to low immediately.
3. Immediately stir in the cheese in batches, starting with the white American cheese. As you stir in the cheese, increase heat to medium/low and whisk CONSTANTLY while the cheese melts. Once each batch is melted/creamy, add more. Don't stop stirring, you have to whisk the entire time while adding cheese.
4. Once done with the white American, add in the shredded fontina or mozzarella. Again, whisk CONSTANTLY while the cheese melts, insuring you have a creamy blend. If you prefer the cheese a bit thicker, add a bit more of the mozzarella.
5. Once all the cheese is melted, stir in the jalapenos, chili powder, nutmeg, red pepper, and salt and pepper. (See note)
6. If you want the queso to be browned like in my pictures, pour the queso into a small nonstick skillet and place in the oven. Broil for 3-4 minutes or until cheese begins to bubble and brown (optional)
7. Top with cilantro, tomatoes, and more jalapenos if desired.
8. Serve with tortilla chips and enjoy!

Prep Time: 35 Minutes

Cook Time: 30 Minutes

Servings: 12

Ingredients

For the Dough:

- 4½ cups bread flour 540 grams
- ⅓ cup granulated sugar 67 grams
- 1 tablespoon instant dry yeast 9 grams
- 1 tablespoon kosher salt 9 grams
- 4 large eggs 230 grams, cold
- 1 large egg yolk 14 grams, cold
- 14 tablespoons whole milk 219 grams, cold (1 cup minus 2 tablespoons)
- 18 tablespoons unsalted butter 254 grams, room temperature, plus more for the pan (2¼ sticks)

For the filling:

- 12 tablespoons unsalted butter 170 grams, melted (1½ sticks)
- 9 tablespoons brown sugar 113 grams (½ cup + 1 tablespoon)
- ¼ cup granulated sugar 50 grams
- 3 tablespoons ground cinnamon 27 grams
- 1 teaspoon pumpkin pie spice 3 grams
- ¼ teaspoon kosher salt
- 1 large egg 50 grams, lightly beaten, for brushing
- 1 tablespoon milk 14 grams, for brushing

For the Icing:

- 2 cups powdered sugar 226 grams
- 6 tablespoons heavy cream 85 grams
- 1 teaspoon pure vanilla extract 4 grams
- ⅛ teaspoon table salt

Instructions

For the Dough:

1. In the bowl of a stand mixer fitted with the dough hook, mix the bread flour, sugar, yeast, and salt on low speed for about 30 seconds.
2. 4½ cups bread flour, ⅓ cup granulated sugar, 1 tablespoon instant dry yeast, 1 tablespoon kosher salt
3. Add eggs and milk and mix until a ball forms around the dough hook, about 4 minutes. Increase the speed to medium and mix until the dough is very smooth, about 5 more minutes.
4. 4 large eggs, 1 large egg yolk, 14 tablespoons whole milk
5. Add the butter, 1 tablespoon at a time, while mixing the dough on medium speed. Incorporate the butter after each addition. It should take about 3 minutes to add all the butter.
6. 18 tablespoons unsalted butter
7. Place the dough in a large, oiled bowl and cover with plastic wrap. Set the bowl in a proofing oven or somewhere warm for the dough to rise, about 1-1½ hours. The dough is very enriched so it may not rise very much.
8. While the dough rises, prepare the filling: Combine the melted butter, brown sugar, granulated sugar, cinnamon, pie spice and salt. The mixture will firm to

a spreadable consistency when kept at room temperature until ready to use. Stir right before using.

9. 12 tablespoons unsalted butter,9 tablespoons brown sugar,¼ cup granulated sugar,3 tablespoons ground cinnamon,1 teaspoon pumpkin pie spice,¼ teaspoon kosher salt

10. Line a baking sheet with parchment. Transfer the dough to the baking sheet and pat it out into a 1-inch-thick rectangle. Cover the dough with plastic wrap.

11. If making the rolls the day of serving, refrigerate the dough for 1 hour or freeze up to 20 minutes. If making the rolls the next day, refrigerate the rolls overnight.

Prep Time: 5 Minutes

Cook Time: 30 Minutes

Servings: 4

Ingredients

- 4 chicken breasts boneless, skinless
- 1 cup Caesar salad dressing
- ½ cup sour cream (optional)
- 1-1½ cup Parmesan cheese grated

Instructions

1. Heat oven to 375F and spray the inside of an 8″ x 11″ baking dish with cooking spray.
2. If the breasts are uneven thickness, pound them (placed in a Ziploc bag and on a flat surface) to an even ¾″-1″ thickness using a meat pounder. Sprinkle the breasts (both sides) with grated Parmesan cheese & freshly ground black pepper, and place them in the prepared baking dish.
3. Whisk together Caesar dressing and sour cream in a small bowl. Pour the Caesar/sour cream mixture over each breasts then sprinkle grated Parmesan cheese on top.
4. Place the prepared chicken in the oven and bake at 375F for 30 minutes or until a meat thermometer inserted in the thickest part of one of the middle breasts reads 150°F.

5. Turn the oven to broil and broil the breasts an additional 2-4 minutes or until the chicken turns golden brown. It can burn quickly, so watch it closely. When done, a meat thermometer should register 165F when stuck into the thickest part of one of the middle breasts. Remove from the oven, cover loosely with foil and allow chicken to rest 5-10 minutes before serving.
6. If desired, garnish with chopped parsley.

Prep Time: 5 Minutes

Cook Time: 30 Minutes

Servings: 4

Ingredients

- 3 tablespoons vegetable oil divided
- 2 large eggs lightly beaten
- 1 pound boneless, skinless chicken breasts cut into small pieces
- 1 cup diced onion
- 1 tablespoon minced garlic 3 cloves
- ½ teaspoon kosher salt
- 3 cups cooked white rice refrigerated
- ½ cup frozen peas and carrots
- 1 ½ tablespoons soy sauce
- 3 green onions thinly sliced
- 1 teaspoon toasted sesame oil

Instructions

1. Heat ½ tablespoon of vegetable oil in a wok (or large nonstick frying pan) over medium-high heat. Add the beaten eggs and gently scramble with a rubber spatula until just softly set, 1-2 minutes. Transfer to a bowl and set aside.
2. 3 tablespoons vegetable oil, 2 large eggs
3. Scrambled eggs in a wok.

4. Add 1 tablespoon of vegetable oil to the wok. Add the chicken, sautéing until lightly brown and fully cooked, about 7 minutes.
5. 1 pound boneless, skinless chicken breasts
6. cooked chicken in a wok.
7. Heat another ½ tablespoon of oil in the wok, and add the onion, garlic, and salt. Cook, stirring occasionally, until the onion is tender, about 4-5 minutes.
8. 1 cup diced onion, 1 tablespoon minced garlic, ½ teaspoon kosher salt
9. cooked chicken in a wok with onion, garlic, and salt.
10. Push the onion mixture to the sides of the wok. Add the remaining 1 tablespoon of vegetable oil and let it heat for a few seconds. Add the cold cooked rice, frozen peas and carrots, and soy sauce. Mix and stir-fry until the rice is heated through, about 3-4 minutes.
11. 3 cups cooked white rice, ½ cup frozen peas and carrots, 1 ½ tablespoons soy sauce
12. Cooked chicken and onions in a wok with frozen peas and carrots and rice.
13. Remove from the heat and stir in scrambled eggs, green onions, and sesame oil. Serve immediately and enjoy!
14. 3 green onions, 1 teaspoon toasted sesame oil
15. Cooked chicken, vegetables, and rice in a wok with scrambled eggs and green onions.

Prep Time: 10 Minutes

Cook Time: 30 Minutes

Servings: 7

Ingredients

- 3 tablespoons unsalted butter
- 2 small shallots peeled and diced
- 4 garlic cloves thinly sliced
- 4 tablespoons all-purpose flour
- ¼ cup dry sherry
- 6 cups chicken stock
- 1 teaspoon kosher salt
- ¼ teaspoon freshly ground black pepper
- 3 sprigs fresh thyme leaves
- 1 bay leaf
- 1½ pounds total white button and cremini mushrooms, coarsely chopped
- ¾ cup half 'n half not milk

Garnish:

- Chopped fresh thyme leaves or parsley
- Sliced fresh sautéed mushrooms
- ¼ cup sliced almonds toasted
- Homemade croutons

Instructions

1. Heat a Dutch oven over medium heat and add the butter. Heat the butter until the bubbling ceases. Add the shallots and cook 2 minutes and add the sliced garlic. Continue cooking until shallots have softened and are translucent, approximately 2 more minutes.
2. Sprinkle the flour over the onion/garlic mixture, stir and cook 1 minute.
3. Stir in the sherry (with a wooden spoon) and scrape the bottom of the pan to deglaze the pan.
4. Add the stock, salt, pepper, bay leaf and thyme sprigs and bring to a boil.
5. Add the mushrooms and bring back to a boil.
6. Reduce the heat to low and simmer, partially covered, for 30 minutes.
7. After 30 minutes, use an immersion blender to purée the soup until smooth and creamy.
8. Add the half 'n half and reheat.
9. If serving immediately, ladle soup into bowls and garnish with chopped fresh parsley and toasted, sliced almonds or homemade croutons.
10. If using as an ingredient in other recipes, remove from the heat and cool to touch. Cover and refrigerate up to 3 days.
11. If freezing the soup for later use, refrigerate the soup (covered) several hours or overnight and divide into quart-size, freezer bags. Keep frozen up to 3 months.
12. Enjoy!

Prep Time: 5 Minutes

Cook Time: 5 Minutes

Servings: 3

Ingredients

- 2 tablespoons brown sugar
- ½ tablespoon paprika
- 1 teaspoon Italian seasoning homemade or store-bought
- ½ teaspoon garlic powder
- ½ teaspoon onion powder
- 1 teaspoon kosher salt
- ¼ teaspoon ground black pepper

Instructions

1. Combine all the ingredients in a small dish.
2. 2 tablespoons brown sugar,½ tablespoon paprika,1 teaspoon Italian seasoning,½ teaspoon garlic powder,½ teaspoon onion powder,1 teaspoon kosher salt,¼ teaspoon ground black pepper
3. combination of spices and seasonings in a small bowl
4. Use as a rub on your favorite cuts of chicken. If using chicken with skin on, be sure to rub some seasoning under the skin as well as on top.
5. mix of spices and seasonings to make a chicken rub

Prep Time: 25 Minutes

Cook Time: 40 Minutes

Servings: 4

Ingredients

- 2 boneless, skinless chicken breasts
- 3 cups buttermilk
- 1 cup all-purpose flour
- 1 tablespoon ground paprika
- 1 tablespoon all-purpose seasoning click link for example
- 1 teaspoon kosher salt
- 1 teaspoon ground black pepper
- 4 tablespoons unsalted butter melted (½ stick)
- ¼ cup fresh flat leaf parsley optional

Instructions

1. CUT chicken breasts in half, lengthwise, to create 4 even portions.
2. 2 boneless, skinless chicken breasts
3. PLACE chicken in a large bowl and marinate in milk for about 20 minutes.
4. 3 cups buttermilk
5. raw chicken breast soaking in buttermilk
6. MIX together flour, paprika, all-purpose spice, salt, and pepper in a medium sized bowl. Set aside.

7. 1 cup all-purpose flour,1 tablespoon ground paprika,1 tablespoon all-purpose seasoning,1 teaspoon kosher salt,1 teaspoon ground black pepper
8. seasoned breading mixture for fried chicken
9. PREHEAT oven to 400°F.
10. Place parchment paper on a 9×13 baking sheet. MELT butter and pour onto the parchment, coating the bottom of the pan/parchment.
11. 4 tablespoons unsalted butter
12. baking tray lined with paper, covered in melted butter
13. Lightly pat each chicken breast with a paper towel to remove excess milk before dipping. DIP each chicken breast, one at a time, in the flour mixture. COAT both sides liberally. PLACE in pan.
14. chicken breast in a bowl, being breaded for fried chicken
15. REPEAT with all four chicken breasts, making sure there is a small amount of room between each breast in the pan. This will allow them to crisp while baking.
16. four pieces of chicken breast covered in flour and breading mixture
17. BAKE at 400°F for 35-40 minutes (or until the breading is golden brown and the juices run clear), flipping each breast after 20 minutes.
18. Remove from oven and transfer to a serving dish. Garnish with parsley if desired. Enjoy!
19. ¼ cup fresh flat leaf parsley

Prep Time: 15 Minutes

Cook Time: 30 Minutes

Servings: 24

Ingredients

For the Dog Treats:

- 2½ cups whole wheat flour 300 grams
- 1 large egg 50 grams
- 1 cup peanut butter 270 grams
- 1 cup water 227 grams
- 2 tablespoons honey 43 grams

For the Frosting:

- 2 tablespoons peanut butter 34 grams
- 1 tablespoon honey 21 grams
- ⅓ cup cornstarch 37 grams (can also use potato starch or arrowroot powder)
- 3-4 tablespoons hot water 43-57 grams

Instructions

1. Preheat oven to 350°F. Line a baking sheet with parchment paper. Set aside.
2. In a large bowl, combine flour and the egg. Add the peanut butter, water, and honey, and stir until you have a stiff dough. The dough becomes very firm and sticky.

You may need to use your hands, or the paddle attachment on your mixer.

3. 2½ cups whole wheat flour,1 large egg,1 cup peanut butter,1 cup water,2 tablespoons honey
4. On a lightly floured surface, roll out the dough about ½-inch thick and use a cookie cutter to make fun shapes. The treats barely spread and rise, so get creative with your shapes.
5. Bake for 18-20 minutes, until golden. Once done, set aside to cool. (If you have smaller cookies, use less time, otherwise the bottom might burn.)
6. To make the frosting, combine the peanut butter and honey in a microwavable bowl, and heat in the microwave in 15 second increments, stirring in between, until melted.
7. 2 tablespoons peanut butter, 1 tablespoon honey
8. Add the melted peanut butter mixture to the cornstarch and stir until just combined.
9. ⅓ cup cornstarch
10. Slowly add in the water 1 tablespoon at a time until you have reached the consistency that you would like. For a thinner frosting, add more water.
11. 3-4 tablespoons hot water
12. Add the frosting to a piping bag and pipe designs on top of each dog treat.
13. Frost the treats with the peanut butter/honey mixture for an even more tempting cookie.

Prep Time: 20 Minutes

Cook Time: 00 Minutes

Servings: 4

Ingredients

- 1 cup fresh blackberries
- 1 cup sugar
- 1 cup water
- 4 sprigs fresh rosemary
- 1 bottle champagne

Instructions

1. In a small saucepan, combine blackberries, sugar, and water. Bring to a boil on high heat, and then reduce to a simmer and let cook for approximately 15-17 minutes. The blackberries will become soft and bright in color and a pinkish purple syrup will form. Making sure it cooks down enough is essential to keeping the ombre effect. Take off of the heat and drain the blackberries, keeping the syrup in a separate bowl. Set both aside and allow to cool.
2. Once blackberries and simple syrup are cooled, spoon about 4 tablespoons of syrup into the bottom of each champagne flute (this recipe makes 4 drinks)
3. Top with champagne.
4. Garnish with fresh blackberries or the cooked blackberries, and a sprig of rosemary.
5. Cheers!

Prep Time: 45 Minutes

Cook Time: 1hr 35 Minutes

Servings: 8

Ingredients

For the Crust:

- 1¼ cups all-purpose flour 150 grams
- 1 teaspoon granulated sugar 4 grams
- ½ teaspoon kosher salt
- ¼ cup unsalted butter 57 grams, COLD and cut into small cubes (½ stick)
- ¼ cup vegetable shortening 46 grams, COLD and cut into cubes (¼ stick – can be larger than the butter)
- ¼ cup ice water 57 grams

For the filling:

- 1¼ pounds sweet potatoes 567 grams (about 3 medium potatoes – you'll need 2 cups mashed)
- 2 large eggs 100 grams
- ½ cup brown sugar 107 grams
- ½ cup granulated sugar 100 grams
- 12 ounces evaporated milk 340 grams (1 can)
- 1 teaspoon pure vanilla extract 4 grams
- ½ teaspoon ground cinnamon
- ½ teaspoon ground nutmeg
- ⅛ teaspoon kosher salt

Instructions

1. In a large bowl, whisk the flour, sugar, and salt together.
2. 1¼ cups all-purpose flour, 1 teaspoon granulated sugar, ½ teaspoon kosher salt
3. Overhead view of dry ingredients for sweet potato pie crust in a glass bowl.
4. Add in the butter and shortening, and a pastry cutter or two forks to combine the ingredients until the butter and shortening are pea-sized pieces or smaller.
5. ¼ cup unsalted butter, ¼ cup vegetable shortening
6. Overhead view of flour with cubes of butter and shortening in a glass bowl.
7. Add in 2 tablespoons of the water and stir until combined. Add the remaining tablespoons, one at a time, until the dough is crumbly, but begins to come together.
8. ¼ cup ice water
9. Overhead view of sweet potato pie dough in a glass bowl.
10. Use your hands to gently knead the dough a few times until it comes together.
11. Turn the dough out onto a piece of plastic wrap and form it into a disc. Wrap tightly and refrigerate for 1 hour.
12. Overhead view of sweet potato pie dough wrapped in plastic wrap.
13. While the dough chills, preheat oven to 425°F. Cut the sweet potatoes in half lengthwise and prick the skin all over. Place them cut-side-down on a parchment-lined baking sheet. Bake until the sweet potatoes are tender all the way through, about 45 minutes.
14. 1¼ pounds sweet potatoes

15. Overhead view of 4 roasted sweet potato halves on a baking sheet.
16. Spray a 9-inch pie plate with nonstick spray.
17. On a floured work surface, roll the chilled pie crust into a 12-inch circle. Transfer it to the pie plate and trim off any excess. Fold the edge of the crust under and use your finger and thumb to shape the crust. Refrigerate while you prepare the filling.
18. Overhead view of sweet potato pie crust pressed into a pie pan and crimped.
19. Once the sweet potatoes are cool enough to touch, scoop out the flesh and add it to a large bowl. Mash it until it is smooth.
20. Overhead view of mashed sweet potato in a glass bowl.
21. Whisk in the eggs until combined.
22. 2 large eggs
23. Overhead view of mashed sweet potato and egg in a glass bowl.
24. Whisk in the brown sugar, sugar, evaporated milk, vanilla extract, cinnamon, nutmeg, and salt until smooth.
25. ½ cup brown sugar,½ cup granulated sugar,12 ounces evaporated milk,1 teaspoon pure vanilla extract,½ teaspoon ground cinnamon,½ teaspoon ground nutmeg,⅛ teaspoon kosher salt
26. Overhead view of sweet potato pie filling in a glass bowl.
27. Pour the filling into the crust and bake for 15 minutes at 425°F.
28. Overhead view of sweet potato pie filling poured into crust in a pie pan.
29. Lower the oven temperature to 350°F and bake for 35-40 minutes, until the crust is golden, the edges of the pie are set, and the center is only slightly jiggly.

30.Overhead view of sweet potato pie in a white pie pan with handles.
31. Let cool completely at room temperature then cover and chill for 2-3 hours before serving.

Prep Time: 15 Minutes

Cook Time: 60 Minutes

Servings: 18

Ingredients

- 2 cups all-purpose flour 240 grams
- 1 teaspoon baking soda 6 grams
- ½ teaspoon baking powder 2 grams
- ½ teaspoon kosher salt
- ½ cup unsalted butter 113 grams, melted (1 stick)
- 6 ripe bananas mashed (about 3 cups or 675 grams)
- ½ cup brown sugar 107 grams
- ¼ cup granulated sugar 50 grams
- 2 large eggs 100 grams, room temperature
- 1 teaspoon pure vanilla extract 4 grams
- ⅓ cup Nutella 90 grams, store-bought or homemade

Instructions

1. Preheat oven to 350°F. Line two 12-count muffin tins with 18 paper liners. Set aside.
2. Overhead view of ingredients for banana nutella muffins.
3. In a medium bowl, whisk the flour, baking soda, baking powder, and salt together. Set aside.
4. 2 cups all-purpose flour, 1 teaspoon baking soda, ½ teaspoon baking powder, ½ teaspoon kosher salt

5. Dry ingredients for banana nutella muffins in a glass bowl next to a half-dozen eggs, a peeled banana, and nutella.
6. Using a hand mixer, beat the butter, bananas, brown sugar, sugar, eggs, and vanilla together on medium speed for 3 minutes. Gently stir in the flour mixture until just combined. Set aside.
7. ½ cup unsalted butter,6 ripe bananas,½ cup brown sugar,¼ cup granulated sugar,2 large eggs,1 teaspoon pure vanilla extract
8. banana nutella muffin batter in a glass bowl next to a half-dozen eggs, a peeled banana, and nutella.
9. Place the Nutella in a small microwave-safe bowl and warm for 30 seconds until it's thinned.
10. ⅓ cup Nutella
11. Fill the wells of the muffin tins so they are ¾ full. Spoon the Nutella over the batter, and swirl them together with a knife.
12. Nutella swirled into banana muffin batter in a muffin tin.
13. Bake for 15-18 minutes, until a toothpick is inserted in the center of the loaf and it comes out clean.
14. Baked banana nutella muffins in a muffin tin.
15. Move the muffins over to a cooling rack and allow them to cool for 15 minutes.

Prep Time: 15 Minutes

Cook Time: 60 Minutes

Servings: 8

Ingredients

For the Meatloaf:

- 1 tablespoon vegetable oil
- 1 yellow onion grated
- 2 cloves garlic minced
- ½ cup Panko breadcrumbs
- ¼ cup whole milk
- 2 large eggs
- 1 teaspoon chopped fresh thyme
- 2 tablespoons Worcestershire sauce
- 1 teaspoon kosher salt
- ¼ teaspoon ground black pepper
- 1 teaspoon garlic powder
- 1 teaspoon onion powder
- 2 pounds 90% lean ground turkey

For the Glaze:

- ¼ cup ketchup
- ¼ cup barbecue sauce store-bought or homemade

Instructions

1. Preheat oven to 350°F. Line a baking sheet with parchment paper or aluminum foil. Set aside.

2. Heat the oil in a sauté pan set over medium-high heat. Once warm, add in the onion and cook until it's translucent, about 3-5 minutes. Add in the garlic and cook until fragrant. Remove from the heat and set aside.
3. 1 tablespoon vegetable oil, 1 yellow onion, 2 cloves garlic
4. sautéing onions in a skillet
5. In a large bowl, whisk the Panko, milk, eggs, thyme, worcestershire, salt, pepper, garlic powder, and onion powder together.
6. ½ cup Panko breadcrumbs,¼ cup whole milk,2 large eggs,1 teaspoon chopped fresh thyme,2 tablespoons Worcestershire sauce,1 teaspoon kosher salt,¼ teaspoon ground black pepper,1 teaspoon garlic powder,1 teaspoon onion powder
7. ingredients in a mixing bowl
8. Add in the onion mixture and turkey. Use your hands to mix until just combined.
9. 2 pounds 90% lean ground turkey
10. ground turkey mixture in a large bowl
11. Transfer the mixture to the baking sheet and pat it into a 9×5-inch loaf.
12. In a medium bowl, whisk the ketchup and barbecue sauce together. Spoon half of the glaze over the meatloaf, spreading it out into an even layer.
13. ¼ cup ketchup, ¼ cup barbecue sauce
14. meatloaf glaze in a small bowl
15. Bake the meatloaf for 40 minutes.
16. Spread the remaining glaze over the meatloaf and bake for another 20 minutes, or until the internal temperature reaches 160°F.
17. glazed meatloaf on a baking tray
18. Cool for 10 minutes before slicing and serving.

Prep Time: 20 Minutes

Cook Time: 60 Minutes

Servings: 4

Ingredients

For the Parker House Rolls:

- ¾ cup warm milk 100-110 degrees F
- 2 teaspoons active dry yeast
- 4 tablespoons butter divided
- 1 large egg
- 2 ½ cups all-purpose flour
- 1 teaspoon kosher salt

For the Ham

- 1 boneless spiral ham about 4 pounds
- ¼ cup light brown sugar
- 1 teaspoon fresh thyme minced
- 1 teaspoon garlic minced

For the Prosciutto Wrapped Asparagus:

- 3 ounces thinly sliced prosciutto about 8 pieces
- ½ pound thick asparagus woody ends trimmed
- 1 teaspoon olive oil

Instructions

For the Parker House Rolls:

1. Add the milk to a medium bowl and sprinkle over the yeast. Set aside for 5 minutes, or until the yeast has bloomed.
2. ¾ cup warm milk,2 teaspoons active dry yeast
3. ingredients for parker house rolls in a white bowl
4. Add two tablespoons of melted butter along with the egg. Whisk to combine.
5. 4 tablespoons butter,1 large egg
6. Add the flour and salt and stir them into the wet ingredients with a dough whisk or wooden spoon.
7. 2 ½ cups all-purpose flour,1 teaspoon kosher salt
8. dough for parker house rolls in a white bowl before rising
9. When a shaggy dough forms, transfer the dough to a clean surface and knead until the dough is smooth- about 2 minutes.
10. Set the dough aside to rise in a warm place until doubled in size– about 1 hour.
11. parker house dinner rolls dough in a white bowl after rising
12. Punch the dough down and roll it into a ½-inch thick rectangle. Cut the dough into rectangles that are approximately 1" wide and 3" long.
13. parker house rolls dough rolled out on a cutting board and sliced
14. Brush the rolls with the remaining melted butter and roll them into circles. Repeat with the remaining pieces of dough.
15. parker house rolls dough rolled out on a cutting board and cut into squares before baking
16. Leave the rolls in a warm place to rise again while you par-bake the ham.

For the Ham:

1. Preheat your oven to 375 degrees F.
2. In a small bowl, combine the brown sugar, thyme, and garlic. Rub the mixture all over the ham.
3. ¼ cup light brown sugar, 1 teaspoon fresh thyme, 1 teaspoon garlic, 1 boneless spiral ham
4. ingredients for brown sugar ham
5. Create a small foil bowl, just large enough to hold the ham. Place the bowl on the sheet pan and then place the ham in the bowl.
6. brown sugar ham on a sheet pan before baking
7. Cover the ham with foil and bake for 30 minutes.
8. For the Prosciutto Wrapped Asparagus
9. Slice the prosciutto in half vertically so you have thin strips.
10. 3 ounces thinly sliced prosciutto
11. ingredients for prosciutto wrapped asparagus
12. Trim the woody ends from the asparagus and wrap each piece with one piece of prosciutto. Set aside until ready to use.
13. ½ pound thick asparagus
14. prosciutto wrapped asparagus spears on a white plate
15. Assembly & Final Bake
16. Once the ham has par baked, create a foil bowl that is large enough to hold all of the rolls– it should be about ¼ the size of your baking sheet.
17. Add the rolls to the bowl and brush the tops with any remaining melted butter.
18. ham and rolls on a sheet pan before baking
19. Bake for another 15 minutes.
20. Finally, add the prosciutto wrapped asparagus to the sheet pan and drizzle them with olive oil.
21. 1 teaspoon olive oil
22. ham, prosciutto wrapped asparagus, and rolls on a sheet pan before baking

23. Bake for a final 10-12 minutes, or until the asparagus is
    tender and the rolls are golden brown.
24. Slice the ham and serve with asparagus and rolls.

Prep Time: 25 Minutes

Cook Time: 1hr 30 Minutes

Servings: 4

Ingredients

For the Turkey Roulade:

- 1 boneless skin-on turkey breast (about 4 pounds)
- 1 cup breadcrumbs
- 3 tablespoons butter melted
- 3 tablespoons olive oil divided
- 1 tablespoon fresh rosemary minced
- 2 teaspoons lemon zest
- 2 cloves garlic minced

For the Sweet Potatoes:

- 2 sweet potatoes peeled and cut into 1" cubes
- 2 teaspoons olive oil
- ½ teaspoon kosher salt
- 1 tablespoon granulated sugar
- ½ teaspoon ground cinnamon

For the Carrots:

- ½ pound small carrots peeled
- 2 teaspoons olive oil
- ½ teaspoon kosher salt
- ½ teaspoon garlic powder
- Fresh chopped parsley for garnish

For the Brussels sprouts:

- ½ pound Brussels sprouts halved
- 2 teaspoons olive oil
- ½ teaspoon kosher salt
- ½ teaspoon fresh thyme minced
- 2 cloves garlic minced

Instructions

For the Turkey Roulade (1.5 hours before serving)

1. Preheat your oven to 325F. Line a large baking sheet with parchment paper.
2. ingredients for turkey roulade
3. Slice the turkey breast in half through the meat (make sure to leave the skin intact) and cover it with plastic wrap. Pound the turkey breast into an even rectangle that is approximately ¾" thick.
4. 1 boneless
5. turkey breast pounded flat between 2 pieces of plastic wrap on a cutting board
6. In a small bowl, combine the breadcrumbs, melted butter, 1 tablespoon olive oil, rosemary, lemon zest, and minced garlic.
7. 1 cup breadcrumbs, 3 tablespoons butter, 3 tablespoons olive oil, 1 tablespoon fresh rosemary, 2 teaspoons lemon zest, 2 cloves garlic
8. Spread the mixture evenly over the turkey.
9. flat turkey breast with breadcrumb mixture on top
10. Beginning with the side without the skin, tightly roll the turkey into a log. You should end up with a tightly rolled turkey, skin side out. Secure the turkey by tying

it with kitchen twine and place it on the parchment lined baking sheet.

11. Drizzle the additional 2 tablespoons of olive oil over the turkey breast and season it generously with salt and pepper. Make sure the olive oil and salt/pepper coat the turkey breast evenly on all sides.
12. rolled up turkey breast with breadcrumb filling on a baking sheet
13. Bake the turkey for 35 minutes, while you prepare the sides.

For the Sweet Potatoes (prepare while the turkey roasts)

1. In a large bowl, combine the sweet potatoes, olive oil, and kosher salt. Toss to combine and set aside until ready to use.
2. 2 sweet potatoes, 2 teaspoons olive oil, ½ teaspoon kosher salt
3. ingredients for roasted sweet potatoes
4. In a small bowl, combine the sugar and cinnamon. Set it aside until ready to garnish.
5. 1 tablespoon granulated sugar, ½ teaspoon ground cinnamon

For the Carrots (prepare while the turkey roasts)

1. In a large bowl, combine the carrots, olive oil, kosher salt, and garlic powder. Mix to combine and set aside until ready to use.
2. ½ pound small carrots, 2 teaspoons olive oil, ½ teaspoon kosher salt, ½ teaspoon garlic powder
3. ingredients for roasted carrots

For the Brussels sprouts (prepare while the turkey roasts)

1. In a large bowl, combine the Brussels sprouts, olive oil, kosher salt, thyme, and garlic. Toss to combine and set aside until ready to use.
2. ½ pound Brussels sprouts, 2 teaspoons olive oil, ½ teaspoon kosher salt, ½ teaspoon fresh thyme, 2 cloves garlic
3. ingredients for roasted Brussels sprouts
4. Final Roast (45 minutes before serving)
5. Remove the turkey breast from the oven and increase the oven temperature to 400F.
6. Add the sweet potatoes, carrots, and brussel sprouts to the pan and roast for 20 minutes.
7. chopped vegetables and turkey roulade on a baking sheet before baking
8. Stir the vegetables and roast for an additional 15 minutes, or until the vegetables are slightly browned and the internal temperature of the turkey registers 165F on an instant read thermometer.
9. chopped vegetables and turkey roulade on a baking sheet after baking
10. Remove the turkey from the oven and cover it with foil. Allow it to rest for 5 minutes.
11. Slice the turkey into ½" slices and serve.
12. Fresh chopped parsley
13. The turkey and vegetables can be kept warm in a 200F for up to 30 minutes.

Prep Time: 30 Minutes

Cook Time: 60 Minutes

Servings: 4

Ingredients

For the Turkey Breast:

- 1 4 pound boneless skin-on turkey breast
- 2 tablespoons butter
- 1 garlic clove minced
- 1 teaspoon fresh rosemary minced
- 1 teaspoon fresh sage minced
- 1 tablespoon olive oil

For the Sweet Potato Casserole:

- 3 large sweet potatoes
- ¼ cup milk
- ¼ cup light brown sugar
- 3 tablespoons butter
- 1 large egg
- 1 teaspoon ground cinnamon
- 1 pinch salt
- 1 cup mini marshmallows

For the Dressing:

- ½ cup chicken stock
- 2 tablespoons butter melted
- 1 large egg
- 1 large carrot chopped

- 1 celery stalk chopped
- 1 shallot chopped
- 2 cloves garlic minced
- 1 teaspoon fresh sage minced
- 4 cups stale bread cubes about 1"

For the Green Beans:

- 1/2 pound green beans
- 1 teaspoon olive oil

Instructions

For the Turkey Breast (1 hour before you plan to eat)

1. Preheat your oven to 400F. Using foil, create a two small bowls that are 1/4 the size of the sheet pan.
2. ingredients for sheet pan turkey breast
3. Pat the turkey breast dry with a paper towel and place it in one of the foil bowls in the baking sheet.
4. 1 4 pound boneless skin-on turkey breast
5. In a small bowl, combine the butter, garlic, rosemary, and sage.
6. 2 tablespoons butter, 1 garlic clove, 1 teaspoon fresh rosemary, 1 teaspoon fresh sage
7. Gently lift the skin away from the meat and place the butter mixture under the skin. Drizzle the olive oil over the outside of the turkey breast and season it with salt and pepper.
8. 1 tablespoon olive oil
9. Roast the turkey for 15 minutes while you prepare the sides.
10. For the Sweet Potatoes (make while the turkey roasts)

11. Poke the sweet potatoes with a fork and par bake them in the microwave for 5 minutes. Test the sweet potatoes by sticking a fork into the center– if it slides in and out easily, they're ready. If not, cook the potatoes for an additional minute and test again.
12. 3 large sweet potatoes
13. ingredients for sweet potato casserole
14. Once the sweet potatoes are soft, carefully split them in half and scrape the flesh into a large bowl.
15. Add the milk, brown sugar, butter, egg, cinnamon, and a pinch of salt. Mix until well combined.
16. ¼ cup milk, ¼ cup light brown sugar, 3 tablespoons butter, 1 large egg, 1 teaspoon ground cinnamon, 1 pinch salt
17. Set aside until ready to use.

For the Dressing (make while the turkey roasts)

1. In a large bowl, whisk together the stock, butter, and egg.
2. ½ cup chicken stock, 2 tablespoons butter, 1 large egg
3. ingredients for turkey dressing
4. Add the carrot, celery, shallot, garlic, and sage. Mix to combine.
5. 1 large carrot, 1 celery stalk, 1 shallot, 2 cloves garlic, 1 teaspoon fresh sage
6. Lastly, add the bread cubes and mix until they are evenly coated. Season with salt and pepper.
7. 4 cups stale bread cubes
8. Set aside until ready to use.
9. Final Roast (45 minutes before you plan to eat)
10. Add the second foil bowl to the sheet pan and place the sweet potatoes inside of it. Top with mini marshmallows.
11. 1 cup mini marshmallows

12. sheet pan dinner with sweet potato casserole, green beans, dressing, and turkey breast before toasting marshmallows
13. Add the dressing to ¼ of the sheet pan, making sure to spread it out in an even layer.
14. Roast the turkey and vegetables for another 15 minutes.
15. Lastly, add the green beans and drizzle with olive oil. Season with salt and pepper, to taste.
16. 1/2 pound green beans,1 teaspoon olive oil
17. Roast for 10 minutes, or until the internal temperature of the turkey registers 165F on an instant read thermometer.
18. Remove the sheet pan from the oven and cover it with foil. Allow the turkey to rest for 10 minutes before slicing.
19. sheet pan dinner with sweet potato casserole, green beans, dressing, and turkey breast
20. This meal can be kept warm in a 200F oven for up to 30 minutes.

Prep Time: 20 Minutes

Cook Time: 1hr 30 Minutes

Servings: 4

Ingredients

For the Maple and Brown Sugar Ham:

- 1 small spiral ham about 5 pounds
- ½ cup brown sugar
- ¼ cup maple syrup
- 2 tablespoons olive oil
- 1 teaspoon minced thyme

For the Scalloped Potatoes:

- 2 large yukon gold potatoes sliced thinly
- ⅓ cup heavy cream
- ½ cup grated parmesan cheese
- 2 garlic cloves minced
- 1 teaspoon fresh parsley minced
- ½ teaspoon kosher salt
- 1 cup grated cheddar cheese

For the Asparagus:

- 1 pound asparagus with the bottom 1-2" removed
- 1 tablespoon olive oil
- 1 teaspoon kosher salt

For the Oven Roasted Deviled Eggs

- 6 large eggs

- 1/4 cup mayonnaise
- 1 tablespoon mustard
- 2 tablespoons pickle relish
- 1 teaspoon kosher salt
- Paprika for garnish

Instructions

1. Par-Bake the Ham
2. Preheat your oven to 350F.
3. In a small bowl, combine the brown sugar, maple syrup, olive oil, and thyme. Add the ham to a large sheet pan and pour over half of the marinade. Cover it with foil. Bake for 1 hour.
4. Make the Scalloped Potatoes (While the Ham is Baking)
5. Combine the potatoes, cream, parmesan, garlic, parsley, and salt in a medium sized microwave safe bowl. Microwave for 5 minutes, or until the potatoes are fork tender. Set aside until ready to use.
6. Make the Asparagus (While the Scalloped Potatoes are Baking)
7. Combine the asparagus, olive oil, and salt in a large bowl and set aside until ready to use.
8. Bake it All Together
9. Remove the foil and top the ham with the remaining sauce.
10. Create a bowl using aluminum foil that is about ¼ of the sheet pan. Add the scalloped potatoes to the bowl and top with grated cheddar cheese.
11. Create another bowl that is about 1/4 the size of the sheet pan and add the eggs to the bowl.

12. Place the scalloped potatoes, eggs, and asparagus on the pan and bake for an additional 35 minutes, or until the ham reaches 140F on an instant read thermometer. Cover the ham with aluminum foil and allow it to rest while you make the deviled eggs.
13. Finish the Deviled Eggs (While the Ham Rests)
14. Remove the eggs from the sheet pan and place them directly into a bowl filled with ice water. Once the eggs are cool to the touch, peel the shells and cut the eggs in half, lengthwise.
15. Remove the yolks and add them to a small bowl with the mayonnaise, mustard, relish, and salt. Stir to combine.
16. Pipe or spoon the mixture back into the egg whites and top with a sprinkle of paprika.

Prep Time: 30 Minutes

Cook Time: 15 Minutes

Servings: 12

Ingredients

- 4 tablespoons vegetable oil 50 grams, divided
- ½ cup ice water 114 grams
- ⅓ cup whole-milk yogurt 76 grams (NOT low or nonfat)
- 1 large egg yolk 14 grams
- 2 cups all-purpose flour 284 grams (10 ounces)
- 1¾ teaspoons granulated sugar 7 grams
- ¾ teaspoon instant or rapid-rise yeast 2 grams
- 3 teaspoons kosher salt 9 grams
- 1½ tablespoons unsalted butter 21 grams, melted

Instructions

1. Brush the inside a large bowl with 1 tablespoon of oil; set aside.
2. 4 tablespoons vegetable oil
3. In a small bowl, combine the ice water, yogurt, remaining 3 tablespoons of oil, and egg yolk. Set aside.
4. ½ cup ice water, ⅓ cup whole-milk yogurt, 1 large egg yolk
5. In a food processor fitted with the metal blade, process the flour, sugar, and yeast just until combined, about 2 seconds.
6. 2 cups all-purpose flour,1¾ teaspoons granulated sugar,¾ teaspoon instant or rapid-rise yeast

7. With the food processor running, slowly add the water/yogurt mixture and process just until no dry flour remains, 10-15 seconds. Now, set the timer and leave the dough alone for 10 minutes.
8. After 10 minutes, add salt to the dough and process 30-60 seconds until dough forms a sticky but satiny ball that just begins to clear the sides of the bowl.
9. 3 teaspoons kosher salt
10. Place the dough on a lightly floured work surface and knead about 2 minutes or until smooth.
11. Shape the dough into a tight ball and place it in the oiled bowl. Roll the dough around the bowl until it is oiled on all sides.
12. Loosely cover the bowl with plastic wrap and place the dough in a proofing oven (at 100°F) or on the countertop at room temperature for 30 minutes.
13. After 30 minutes, fold the partially risen dough up and over itself 8 times (gently lift and fold the edge of dough toward the middle of the dough ball), tuning the dough 90 degrees with each fold. Re-cover the bowl with plastic wrap and let rise another 30 minutes.
14. Repeat the folding, turning, rising one more time. When done, there should be three 30-minute rises.
15. Transfer the dough to a lightly floured work surface and divide into 12 equal portions (they don't need to be rounded). My portions usually end up rectangular or triangular in shape.
16. Place the dough portions on a lightly oiled baking sheet and let stand 15-30 minutes until slightly raised and are a little puffy(ish).
17. Adjust oven rack to middle position and preheat oven to 350°F while the rolls proof/rest.
18. Brush the dough with melted butter and sprinkle with salt, if desired.

19. 1½ tablespoons unsalted butter
20. Bake at 350°F for 15-25 minutes or until light golden brown and the internal temperature registers between 201°F-205°F.
21. Transfer tray to a cooling rack and serve while warm and fresh.

21. Italian Sausage Sheet Pan Dinner

Prep Time: 10 Minutes

Cook Time: 40 Minutes

Servings: 6

Ingredients

- ½ pound green beans topped and tailed
- 2 cups carrots cut into ½ inch chunks
- 3 cups baby white potatoes cut into ½ inch chunks
- 1 red bell pepper cut into ½ inch chunks
- 3 tablespoons olive oil
- ½ tablespoon minced garlic
- 1 ½ teaspoons Italian spice
- 1 teaspoon oregano
- ½ teaspoon salt
- ½ teaspoon ground black pepper
- 4 Italian sausage links cut into coins 1 inch thick
- Fresh parsley for garnish

Instructions

1. Preheat oven to 400F.
2. Line a sheet pan with aluminum foil or parchment paper. Set aside.
3. Place the carrots, potatoes and pepper chunks into a large bowl.
4. Drizzle with olive oil and add the garlic, Italian spice, oregano, salt and pepper. Toss to coat.

5. Use a slotted spoon to transfer the vegetables onto the sheet pan. Spread them out evenly.
6. Put the green beans in the bowl the other vegetables came out of and toss them to coat them in the remaining oil and spices. Set aside.
7. Place the sausage coins on the sheep pan in amongst the vegetables.
8. Bake for 25 minutes. Remove from the oven mix in the green beans and return to the oven for an additional 15 minutes.
9. Garnish with fresh chopped parsley.

Prep Time: 10 Minutes

Cook Time: 25 Minutes

Servings: 6

Ingredients

- 2 pounds Jumbo raw shrimp peeled and deveined
- 16 ounces fresh broccoli about 2 heads
- 2 Tablespoons olive oil
- Salt and pepper to taste

For the sauce:

- ½ cup honey
- ¼ cup soy sauce
- 1 Tablespoon lemon juice
- 4 teaspoons minced garlic
- 1 teaspoon ginger paste
- 2 teaspoons sesame seeds
- 3 teaspoons equal parts cornstarch and water
  Suggested side:
- Brown rice

Instructions

1. Preheat oven to 400F and line a sheet pan with silicone baking mat or parchment paper.
2. In a small bowl, mix together ingredients for the sauce, except for cornstarch and water.
3. Wash broccoli then chop into bite sized florets.

4. Prepare shrimp by mixing with ½ of the sauce mixture. Toss to coat and cover to marinate until broccoli is done.
5. Spread broccoli on prepared sheet pan then drizzle with olive oil. Toss by hand to coat then salt and pepper to taste.
6. Roast in oven on middle rack for 15 minutes.
7. Move roasted broccoli to one side of the pan and place shrimp on the other side.
8. Place sheet pan back in the oven and cook for an additional 8-10 minutes. Shrimp are done when they curl into a "C" shape and are pink in color.
9. Combine cornstarch and water, set aside.
10. While sheet pan is completing the final cook time, heat remaining sauce to a simmer, add cornstarch mixture then stir well until reduced to a thicker sauce.
11. Plate and drizzle sauce.
12. ENJOY an easy clean up!

Prep Time: 15 Minutes

Cook Time: 15 Minutes

Servings: 4

Ingredients

For the Herb Lamb Chops:

- 1 rack Frenched Lamb Chops see notes
- 1 tablespoon olive oil
- 2 garlic cloves minced
- 1 teaspoon minced sage leaves
- 1 teaspoon minced thyme leaves

For theSmashed Potatoes:

- 1 pound miniature potatoes
- 1 tablespoon olive oil
- 1 teaspoon kosher salt

For the Rainbow Carrots:

- 4-6 large or 10-12 small rainbow carrots
- 1 teaspoon olive oil
- ½ teaspoon kosher salt

For theGreen Beans:

- 1 pound green beans ends trimmed
- 1 teaspoon olive oil
- ½ teaspoon kosher salt

Instructions

For the Lamb Chops:

1. Preheat your oven to 425F. Score the fat cap of the lamb chops in a crosshatch pattern and season it generously with salt and pepper.
2. In a small bowl, combine the olive oil, garlic, sage, and thyme. Rub the mixture over the lamb and set it aside to marinate while you make the sides.

For the Smashed Potatoes:

1. Bring a large pot of salted water to a boil. Add the potatoes and cook for 12-14 minutes, or until the potatoes are fork tender.
2. Remove the potatoes from the water and pat them dry on a towel (be careful, they're hot). Gently smash the potatoes with a potato masher (or the flat side of a cup). Place the smashed potatoes on the sheet pan (try to make sure they don't take up more than ¼ of the sheet pan) and drizzle them with olive oil and sprinkle with salt.
3. Bake for 10 minutes while you prepare the other sides.

For the Roasted Carrots:

1. Combine the carrots, olive oil, and salt in a small bowl and set aside until ready to use.

For the Green Beans:

2. Combine the green beans, olive oil, and salt in a small bowl and set aside until ready to use.
3. Roast It All Together

4. Add the carrots and green beans to the sheet pan, making sure it's not overcrowded– if it is, you may need to use two sheet pans.

5. Wrap the exposed bones of the lamb with aluminum foil and place it fat side up on the sheet pan. Bake for 15 minutes, then turn the heat down to 350F and bake for an additional 10 minutes, or until your desired doneness.

6. Remove the sheet pan from the oven and cover it with foil. Allow the lamb to rest for 10 minutes before slicing.

Prep Time: 15 Minutes

Cook Time: 25 Minutes

Servings: 4

Ingredients

- 4 skinless, boneless chicken breasts halves
- 2 tbsp olive oil
- 1 teaspoon coarse sea salt
- 1 teaspoon paprika

Instructions

1. Preheat oven to 400 degrees F
2. Rub chicken breasts with olive oil and sprinkle both sides with salt and paprika. Then place chicken in a broiler pan.
3. Bake chicken breasts at 400 degrees for 10 minutes.
4. Flip chicken and cook another 15 minutes, until no longer pink in the center and the juices are clear. An instant-read thermometer inserted into the center should read at least 165 degrees F
5. Serve immediately alongside vegetables, potatoes, or your favorite side dish!

Prep Time: 30 Minutes

Cook Time: 10 Minutes

Servings: 12

Ingredients

- 2 cups boiling water
- 1½ cups 12 tablespoons shortening
- 2/3 cup granulated sugar
- 2 teaspoons salt
- 2 teaspoons kosher salt
- 2 1/4 oz. envelopes active dry yeast
- ½ cup warm water 105° - 115°
- 2 eggs lightly beaten
- 7½-8 cups all-purpose flour
- ½ cup butter divided and melt

Instructions

1. Place the shortening, sugar and salt in the bowl of a stand mixer. Pour the boiling water over all. Stir on low until shortening melts and the sugar and salt have dissolved. Let stand until the mixture registers 110°F.
2. In a 1-cup measuring cup, combine yeast and warm water. Be sure water is between 105°F-115°F. Stir with a fork approximately 10 times and let stand 5 minutes.
3. Add the yeast mixture and lightly beaten eggs to the shortening mixture, and beat on low until combined. Add the flour, ¼ cup at-a-time, while mixer is on low speed. This should take 2-3 minutes. Dough is ready

when it begins to pull away from the sides of the bowl. Dough should be very soft and smooth.

4. Place the dough in a large, lightly greased mixing bowl. Turn the dough over in the bowl, so all sides are greased. Cover the bowl with plastic wrap and refrigerate 8-24 hours.

5. When ready to use, place the amount of dough needed on a floured surface. (Cover any remaining dough with plastic wrap and keep refrigerated up to 24 hours, total.) Knead the removed dough until smooth and elastic, approximately 2 minutes.

6. Lightly grease a muffin pan. Shape dough into 1-inch balls. Dip each ball into melted butter then place in a muffin cups. Place three balls, side-by-side, into each muffin cup.

7. Cover rolls loosely with plastic wrap or clean (lightweight) dishtowel. Allow dough to rise in a warm place (85°F-100°F works best), until double in size (approximately 45-60 minutes).

8. Preheat oven to 400°F. If desired, sprinkle rolls very lightly with flake sea salt (like Maldon's). Bake rolls 8-12 minutes or until golden brown. Brush with remaining butter and serve immediately.

Prep Time: 15 Minutes

Cook Time: 10 Minutes

Servings: 4

Ingredients

- 2 tablespoons butter
- 3 cloves garlic finely minced
- 2 tablespoons tomato paste
- 1 teaspoon Italian seasoning
- ½ teaspoon salt
- ½ teaspoon ground black pepper
- ½ cup vodka
- ½ cup pasta water
- 1 cup heavy cream
- 2 cups freshly grated parmesan cheese
- 12 ounces penne pasta cooked

Instructions

1. Melt the butter in a large skillet over medium heat then add the garlic and cook until it becomes fragrant, about one minute.
2. 2 tablespoons butter,3 cloves garlic
3. Add the tomato paste, Italian seasoning, salt and pepper and stir and cook until the tomato paste becomes fragrant, about 1 minute.
4. 2 tablespoons tomato paste,1 teaspoon Italian seasoning,½ teaspoon salt,½ teaspoon ground black pepper

5. Pour in the vodka and pasta water and stir and cook until it starts to thicken then add the heavy cream and stir and cook once again before adding the parmesan cheese, stirring until it melts.
6. ½ cup vodka,½ cup pasta water,1 cup heavy cream,2 cups freshly grated parmesan cheese
7. mixing cheese into the sauce
8. Add the pasta and stir once again then serve with freshly minced parsley for garnish if desired.
9. 12 ounces penne pasta
10. penne pasta being mixed into the vodka sauce

Prep Time: 10 Minutes

Cook Time: 15 Minutes

Servings: 6

Ingredients

- 1 pound cavatappi pasta
- 2 tablespoons unsalted butter
- 2 cloves garlic minced
- 8 ounces basil pesto
- ½ teaspoon salt
- ½ cup heavy cream
- Grated Parmesan cheese and fresh basil for serving

Instructions

1. Cook the pasta until al dente according to package directions. Reserve ½ cup of the pasta water. Drain the noodles and set them aside.
2. 1 pound cavatappi pasta
3. boiling pasta in a pot
4. While the pasta cooks, melt the butter in a skillet over medium heat. Add the garlic and cook until fragrant, about 30 seconds.
5. 2 tablespoons unsalted butter, 2 cloves garlic
6. Stir in the pesto and salt and cook until the pesto starts to bubble, about 1-2 minutes.
7. 8 ounces basil pesto, ½ teaspoon salt
8. Pour in the reserved pasta water. Stir and cook until the sauce begins to thicken, about 5 minutes.

9. Reduce the heat to low, pour in the heavy cream, stir, and let it simmer until it reduces a bit, about 2-3 minutes.
10. ½ cup heavy cream
11. Add the pasta and toss to coat. Serve with Parmesan cheese and basil.
12. Grated Parmesan cheese and fresh basil
13. pesto covered pasta in a large pot

Prep Time: 10 Minutes

Cook Time: 10 Minutes

Servings: 6

Ingredients

- 1 tablespoon sesame oil
- 3 green onions sliced, divided
- 3 cloves garlic minced
- 8 ounces cremini mushrooms sliced
- 8 ounces fresh snap peas
- 1 red bell pepper julienned
- 1 carrot julienned
- 8 ounces dry lo mein egg noodles see note
- Sesame seeds optional, for garnish
- 0 Mein Sauce
- 3 tablespoons low-sodium soy sauce see note
- ½ tablespoon mirin
- 1 teaspoon brown sugar
- 1 teaspoon toasted sesame oil
- ½ teaspoon ground ginger
- ¼ teaspoons crushed red pepper flakes optional

Instructions

1. In a small bowl, whisk together the lo mein sauce ingredients and set aside.
2. ½ tablespoon mirin,1 teaspoon brown sugar,1 teaspoon toasted sesame oil,½ teaspoon ground

ginger,¼ teaspoons crushed red pepper flakes,3 tablespoons low-sodium soy sauce

3. Heat the sesame oil in a wok or large skillet set over medium high heat. Add half of the green onions and garlic, cooking for 30 seconds until fragrant.
4. 1 tablespoon sesame oil,3 green onions,3 cloves garlic,8 ounces cremini mushrooms,8 ounces fresh snap peas,1 red bell pepper,1 carrot
5. Green onions and garlic cooking in oil in a wok.
6. Stir in the mushrooms, snap peas, bell pepper, and carrot. Cook, stirring frequently, until tender, 4-5 minutes.
7. Vegetables added to a wok.
8. Meanwhile, in a large pot of boiling water, cook and drain the noodles according to package instructions.
9. 8 ounces dry lo mein egg noodles
10. Stir in cooked noodles and sauce mixture and toss to combine. Serve immediately, garnished with remaining green onions and sesame seeds.
11. Sesame seeds
12. Overhead view of vegetable lo mein in a wok.

Prep Time: 10 Minutes

Cook Time: 15 Minutes

Servings: 8

Ingredients

- 1 ½ pounds lean ground beef
- 1 cup onion diced
- 1 green pepper diced
- 4 cloves garlic minced
- 14.5 ounces diced tomatoes 1 can
- 14.5 ounces crushed tomatoes 1 can
- 15 ounces tomato sauce 1 can
- 2 cups beef broth
- 1 tablespoon Worcestershire sauce
- 1 ½ teaspoons Italian seasoning
- 1 teaspoon kosher salt
- ½ teaspoon paprika
- ½ teaspoon ground black pepper
- 16 ounces macaroni noodles
- Shredded cheddar cheese for serving

Instructions

1. Heat the Instant Pot using the Sauté-Normal function. Add the ground beef, onion, and green pepper, cooking the beef until it's no longer pink. Remove any excess grease.

2. 1 ½ pounds lean ground beef, 1 cup onion, 1 green pepper

3. Press Cancel and stir in the minced garlic. Add the diced tomatoes, crushed tomatoes, tomato sauce, broth, Worcestershire sauce, Italian seasoning, paprika, salt, and pepper. Stir well to combine.

4. 4 cloves garlic,14.5 ounces diced tomatoes,14.5 ounces crushed tomatoes,15 ounces tomato sauce,2 cups beef broth,1 tablespoon Worcestershire sauce,1 ½ teaspoons Italian seasoning,1 teaspoon kosher salt,½ teaspoon paprika,½ teaspoon ground black pepper

5. mixing ingredients in a pressure cooker

6. Add the macaroni noodles and press them down so they're submerged underneath the liquid. Attach the Instant Pot lid. Ensure the valve is in the "sealing" position.

7. 16 ounces macaroni noodles

8. Set the Instant Pot to Pressure Cook – Manual for 5 minutes. Perform a quick pressure release when the timer goes off.

9. Carefully remove the lid and stir the goulash. Serve topped with shredded cheddar cheese.

Prep Time: 10 Minutes

Cook Time: 5hrs 2 Minutes

Servings: 8

Ingredients

- 1 pound dried black-eyed peas
- 7 cups low-sodium chicken broth store-bought or homemade
- 14 ounces diced tomatoes (1 can)
- 1 cup fully-cooked diced smoked sausage beef, pork, turkey, or a blend
- 1 onion diced
- 1 stalk celery diced
- 1 jalapeño pepper diced
- 4 cloves garlic minced
- 1 bay leaf
- 2 sprigs fresh thyme
- 2 teaspoons cajun seasoning
- ½ teaspoon ground black pepper
- Kosher salt to taste

Instructions

1. To a large crockpot, add all the ingredients except the salt. Stir to combine.
2. 1 pound dried black-eyed peas,7 cups low-sodium chicken broth,14 ounces diced tomatoes,1 cup fully-cooked diced smoked sausage,1 onion,1 stalk celery,1

jalapeño pepper,4 cloves garlic,1 bay leaf,2 sprigs fresh thyme,2 teaspoons cajun seasoning,½ teaspoon ground black pepper

3. Ingredients for crockpot black eyed peas in a crockpot.
4. Cover and cook on high for 5-6 hours.
5. Crockpot black eyed peas in a crockpot.
6. Remove the bay leaf, add salt to taste, and serve!